I0464940

THOUGHTS WITHOUT THINKING

TAKING CONTROL OVER YOUR RACING THOUGHTS

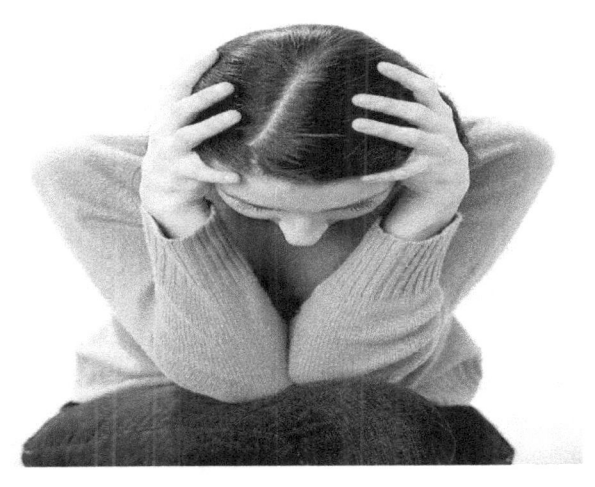

By Patricia A. Carlisle

Introduction

I want to thank you and congratulate you for choosing the book, **"THOUGHTS WITHOUT THINKING: Taking control over your racing thoughts"**.

This book contains proven steps and strategies on how to take control over your thoughts.

The vast majority consider anxiety the cause of fearful or uncertain thoughts. In any case, it is not generally just the frightful thoughts are the issue. A few individuals experience racing thoughts, where it feels as if their brain is going hundred miles per hour. At times, those thoughts are frightful. If those thoughts are infrequent, and rare that's not considered a problem.

Yet, when you have racing thoughts it can be exceptionally upsetting, which is the reason it is critical to discover individual approaches to control racing thoughts. In this book you will discover the most practical ways to approach racing thoughts, and stop them from taking control over your life.

Thanks again for choosing this book, I hope you enjoy it!

TABLE OF CONTENT

Chapter 9

MINDFUL BREATHING

Preview Of 'Coping with Anxiety Disorder: How to stop anxiety tension.'

Chapter 1

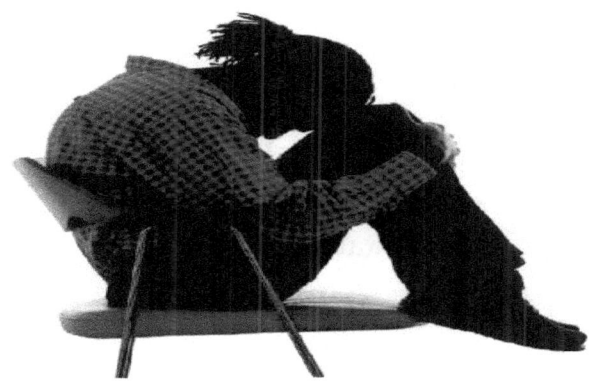

RACING THOUGHTS

Racing thoughts are a strange issue. It's not simply the substance of the idea, it's the way it feels as if your thoughts are firing at such a quick pace to the point that you can't considerably recall what the last thought was. And when you have another thought another instantly takes its place.

Racing thoughts may influence anybody with anxiety, however, it is most common for those who have anxiety attacks. Racing thoughts might like wise influence those with summed up anxiety issues that may influence anybody when they encounter anxiety.

It's likewise extremely common at sleep for reasons unknown, numerous individuals discover that their thoughts appear to be quicker when they're attempting to get to sleep. And shockingly, when they happen at mid bedtime, it can be difficult to get any sleep. The reasons for racing thoughts are likely identified with the way your neurotransmitters interface aid anxiety, alongside the surge of adrenaline you get when you have anxiety (which may make your mind significantly more dynamic). Adrenaline, particularly, causes your psyche to be over-dynamic while at the same time making it harder to core interest. Different reasons may include:

1) One of the reason may happen when your attempting to go to bed, is on the count of there are no distractions. When you're left with your own thoughts, your thoughts frequently go unchecked, and in the end they are untamed.

2) Anxiety might also bring about hyperventilation, which can incidentally bring about less blood stream to the cerebrum. This is particularly common when experiencing an anxiety attack. It's likely that your mind is really not working, and you're having difficulty stopping the thoughts. Try not to stress- this isn't risky.

3) Lack of sleep is the main reason behind this. Anxiety can also stop you from sleeping, and the lack of sleep may also prompt racing thoughts. This can often become a self-satisfying issue, since anxiety prompts absence of rest, which prompts racing thoughts, which prompts an absence of rest. That is why most people seem to experience repeated thoughts, and it becomes extremely upsetting.

Chapter 2

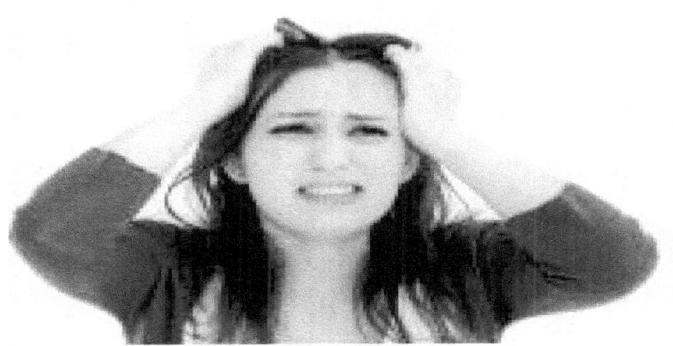

REASONS FOR RACING THOUGHTS

There isn't a clear "reason" for racing thoughts. It is probable that anxiety causes your brain to both respond all the more rapidly while limiting your ability to control those thoughts, and you are unable to concentrate.

Keep in mind that anxiety should be looked at as your emergency call of your "fight or flight" system, a system that should keep you safe from threat. Thinking excessively rapidly is really boosting your protection, and not concentrating a lot on any given thought may be an advantage. It guarantees a speedy response. In any case, since you have an anxiety issue where no apprehensions are available it is not uncommon for racing thoughts to be up setting, and may even prompt more anxiety.

Racing thoughts aren't an indication of any danger; however they are clearly a critical issue. They make it difficult to focus, and without focus it is difficult to adapt to anxiety. This is the reason it is so important to stop your racing thoughts. The arrangement have the tendency to contract a bet of relying on a thought when your racing thoughts happen. They for the most part, happen at 3 times.

1. During the height of an anxiety attack.

2. When your are attempting to go to sleep.

3. For no reason at all when you have anxiety.

We should break out a few tips for controlling your racing thoughts taking into account when they happen.

Chapter 3

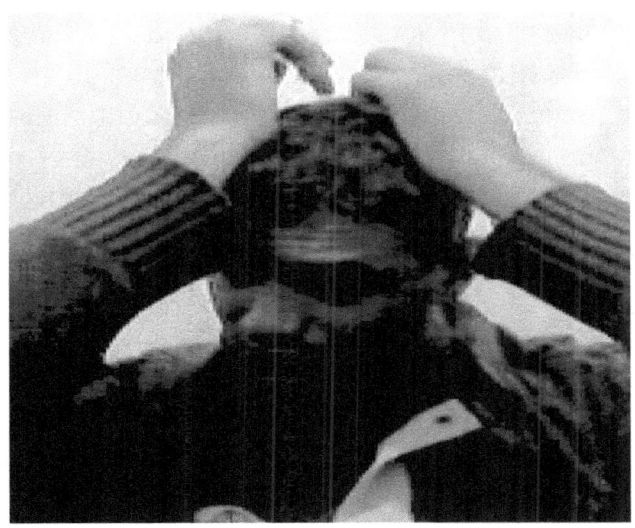

PANIC ATTACKS AND RACING THOUGHTS

In the middle of a panic attack, your thoughts are frequently racing, and health related. You pay consideration on every single change in your body, thinking of what's going on, and and frequently encounter this level of perplexity that just aggravate your thoughts.

Your objective is to basically attempt to take yourself out of your own head. You can't stop the adrenaline that pumps through your brain when you are encountering an anxiety attack; however, you can use coping skills that will help make the racing thoughts less annoying, and possibly fight the anxiety that causes them. A few methods include:

1) Distractions are a key part for curing racing thoughts. They're really a necessary one. You have to learn how to occupy your brain from itself, so your racing

thoughts don't turn out to be excessively extreme. This is what "escape from your own head," mean having to do something like calling someone that knows you have panic attacks, and talking with them. Talking on the telephone removes a great deal of your thoughts, and also reduces the measure of consideration you give to your anxiety, as a result, reducing your racing thoughts.

2) Hyperventilation is one of the conceivable reasons for racing thoughts. Since it causes a dizziness which makes it harder to concentrate. You can decrease this by backing off your breathing so your carbon dioxide levels increase. Try not to hold your breath, yet do take moderate, controlled breaths, and battle any desire to over-relax.

3) Meditation has long been advertize as a relaxing method, yet for those with racing personalities it might be particularly helpful. You can also listening to music to calm the brain. Mantras are lengthened sounds that cause your neck to vibrate. Close your eyes, and begin singing a song while breathing gradually, and you may be able to take control of your thoughts until they slow down.

Panic attacks regularly need to run their course before they can be completely controlled, on the grounds if your panic attack by it extreme nature is a temporary loss of control. In any case, the above methods will help you to return to your ordinary speed of thought. And after that, when the panic attack passes you can return to your ordinary life.

Chapter 4

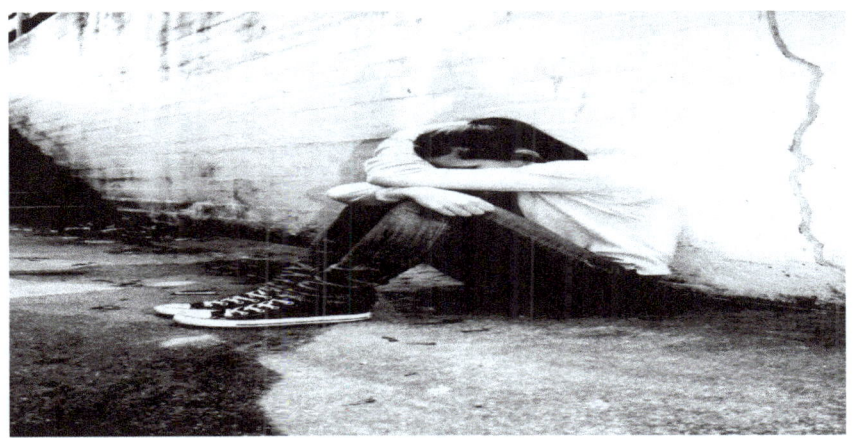

ANXIETY AND RACING THOUGHTS

Anxiety and racing thoughts when you're attempting to sleep can be extremely distracting, and shockingly, they have a tendency to expand on themselves bring about more major anxiety that winds up keeping you awake. I ask a lot of people what makes them stay alert during evening, and it is not generally fear. It is normally an inclination that they can't turn off their mind.

Not everyone experiences negative thoughts. Some experience a personality that doesn't have a sensible focus, despite the fact the thoughts themselves are harmless. This may not even by created by anxiety, however tragically those with anxiety have a tendency to react to racing thoughts with more stress and anxiety, which still makes it harder to sleep. Consider the below coping technique:

1) **Write out the Thoughts**- It began by attempting to work out any of these thoughts on some kind paper or diary. The mind tries to make it difficult to recall

things, particularly before sleeping. The brain additionally doesn't stress over remembering things when it knows you made a note of them. Racing thoughts may happen when your brain is attempting to recall the thoughts you are trying to keep track of, so write them out on a paper to give your mind some relief it will help you unwind.

2) **Get Up and Do Something**-Your racing thoughts will develop not just by your anxiety. Racing thoughts can develop when you're relaxed, and attempting to fall asleep. In the event that you discover that your mind began to race, try to find something to keep you busy. Soon you'll see that all you needed was a distraction, and you will start to think of something to do each time as a tool to guarantee that you will be relaxed when you attempt to go to sleep later.

3) **Distracting White Noise**-Many individuals utilize what's known as "white noise" as a sort of mental distraction. It's a different type of tangible distraction. When your mind is being occupied by a sound, it can't concentrate as much on its thoughts. For example, listening to something like a talk radio at a low volume so you can barely make out the words. This will give your psyche something else it needs to focus on so your thoughts can't be as active.

Chapter 5

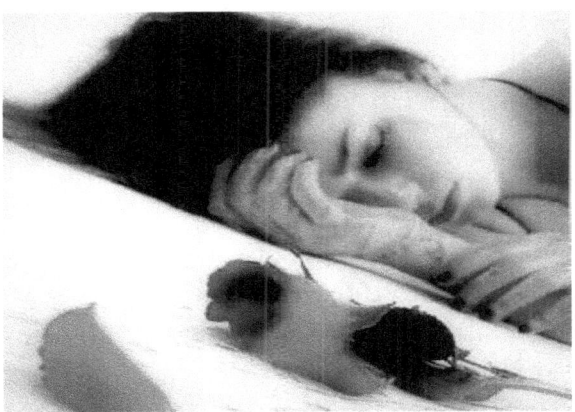

SLEEP, ANOTHER CURE

Sleep is additionally its own particular cure. In the event that you can locate a couple of days to attempt to make up any lack of sleep you may have, you'll frequently find that your mind don't race as much as it use to. At long last, what will be advisable for you to do when you thoughts don't appear to race for any genuine reason other than gentle or day by day anxiety. This is the point at which you appear to have racing thoughts now and again at no particular time regularly regardless of you encounter anxiety.

Also it's hard to call anxiety the reason for your racing thoughts. Yet, you're not so much miss an anxiety attack. If this is the case, you might have to resource into some different tactics in order to help control your racing thoughts. Consider the ideas listed below.

Exercise/Jog-Jogging is an exceptional way for tiring the brain. Wellness doesn't simply tire muscles. It makes your mind more relaxed as well, by releasing chemicals that give an unwinding/quieting impact. So practicing and/or going for a run is profitable.

1) **Walking**-If you can't work out, walk. Walking gives a lot of physical distraction. It gives you the opportunity to enjoy new sights, sounds, and smells, and gives you an even blood flow that will help quiet your body and mind.

2) **Give yourself a task**-Find something you can accomplish as your mind continues to race. Activities give you something to concentrate on. Try not to stress a lot over your thoughts racing, because if you attempt to stop it, you can make it worse. Rather, give yourself something to do that focus your mind on something that does not require as much thought, such as making up for lost time with your friends and family.

Chapter 6

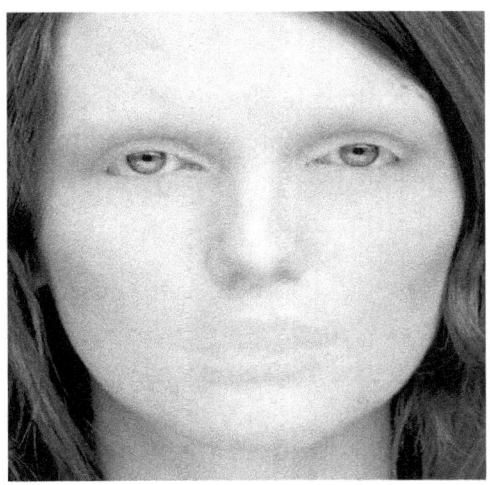

JUST SAY "STOP IT"

There are a varieties of methods of controlling caring thoughts by just instructing yourself to say "stop it". For it to work successfully, you'd need to practice it, stand in front of your mirror and tell yourself to stop it. This can be encouraging.

The "stop it" system is an intellectual behavioral treatment utilized by therapist to influence the negative thinking in individuals. The stop procedure is not obviously the only thing you can do to stop racing thoughts.

Racing thoughts can also be control by just captivating your mind. When your brain is completely drawn in it makes it harder for thoughts to rise up to the top, and command your attention. Here is some suggestion you can do to stop racing thoughts in their track:

1) **Talk with someone, or better yet to a few individuals**. Getting into discussion is the best distraction on the planet. It takes a considerable

amount of intellectual skills to hold a conversation, and this will help you forget about what you were thinking about at that time.

2) **Read a book**. This is valuable because it has a tendency to possess your inward voice. So if you are following the story it is a great deal harder to slip into a different thoughts in the mean time.

3) **Composing**. Whether it is a diary, website, music, or journaling; the expression of composing will draw in your psyche and reduce the force of racing thoughts.

CHAPTER 7

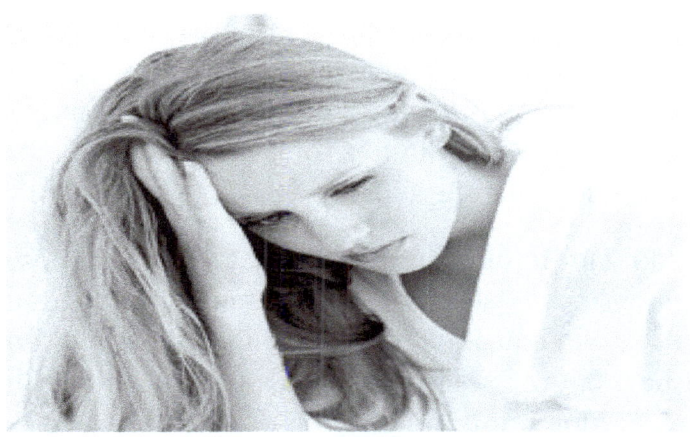

HAVING RACING THOUGHTS DOES NOT MEAN YOU'RE CRAZY OR INSANE

Having racing thoughts can be aggravating, and terrifying because it can make you feel like you are crazy. Yet, having racing thoughts does not mean you're crazy or insane. It does imply that you are on edge, and that your anxiety level is rise. Anxiety and racing thoughts simply go hand and hand.

Most individuals do not know our everyday activities can be the root cause of our mental disturbance. When you feel your mind is racing, it is advised that we began by take your foot of the accelerator.

A few of us have a large amount of things that we take care of in our lives. Each waking moment of our day is filled with activities, and we never have time to rest. Everyone needs to be productive because it gives us a feeling of achievement and reason. The issue with having an excess of responsibilities is that all the activities stimulate our minds so much that it turns out to be progressively harder to relax.

To address this issue, it is recommended to make a note of every activity and responsibility, including reflection. Keep in mind that your spiritual advancement is critical to your family's happiness; it will empower you to really be there for them. At that point, organize your duties to add family's pleasures, and set aside a few minutes for your own needs for example, rest and reflection.

With a considerably lot in our duties, we must learn to choose between options. We can't stop our employments or abandon our families, yet we can consider carefully what we really need to survive and be content. Ask yourself, do all your material things truly make your family happy, or do they detract us from our friends and family?

Chapter 8

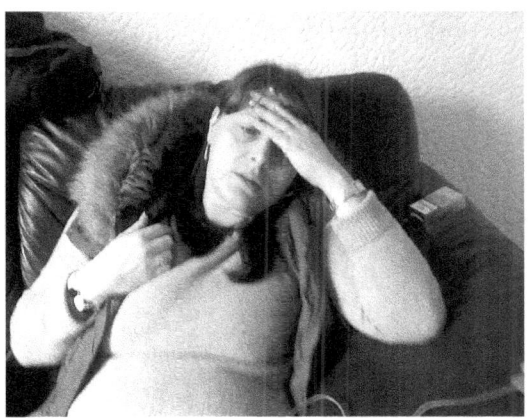

BACKGROUND NOISE

Background noise is another mental disturbance, and most of it is pointless. When we're driving home after work, we'll turn on the radio in our car to help us loosen up, at the same time, we think about work or things we have to do at home, for example, keeping an eye on the children or making supper.

When we return home, we may turn on the TV while we settle in, not paying attention to what's on. We typically do this unknowingly to overcome the steady chatter in our mind. What we may not understand it is disturbing our mind much more, and when it does not work, we may present ourselves with a beverage to help us unwind.

A few individuals turn on the radio or TV while they work, because they feel this helps them focus. The reason this appears to help is because the additional sound keeps uncomfortable thoughts from rising to the surface, yet the background noise just makes more noise.

Obviously, we should utilize some judgment concerning what we watch, or listen to on TV or the radio. Keep in mind, whatever seeds in your mind you water, those will be the ones that develop.

It is recommended that turning off the radio or TV when you're doing something else. This will help you focus on what you're doing. Attempt it for a week; you'll be amazed at what a difference it will make.

Chapter 9

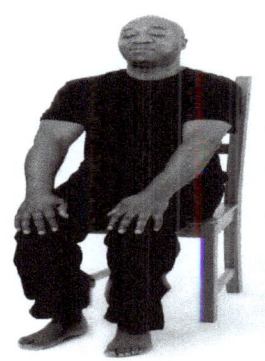

MINDFUL BREATHING

Mindful breathing is a basic tool for keeping your mind from racing thoughts. Rehearsing "mindful breathing" is simple, and doesn't take long; it will help with the thoughts in your mind. This will empower you to think with more clarity, since you'll have less mental activity.

You should simply stop, and take some time in your day to take three to five "mindful breaths". You don't need to put a strain on your chest to focus on your breathing just relax, but instead simply pay attention to how you are breathing. Mindful breathing additionally has different advantages. It gives us time to reflect on are goals and achievements while breathing, and it takes us back to the present moment, which is the place where truth is reality. You may need to post a reminder note some place where you will see it for the duration of the day because it is too important to overlook you mindful breathing.

Considering above facts it is clear that controlling your racing thoughts is an uphill battle, but not a battle that you cannot win. It's basically in your hands to practice controlling your racing thoughts, and achieving your goals.

Conclusion

Thank you again for choosing this book!

I hope this book was able to give you ideas on how to stop hearing voices.

The next step is to try the techniques in this book.

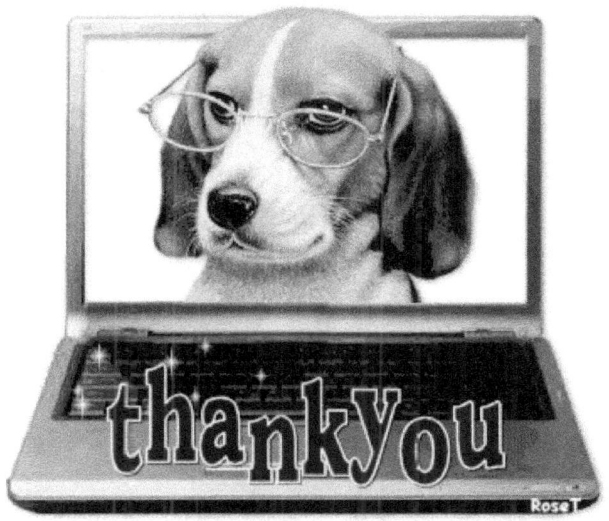

Finally, if you enjoyed this book would you be kind enough to leave a review for this book on Amazon? It'd be greatly appreciated!

Leave a review for this book on Amazon.com!

Thank you and good luck!

Preview Of 'Coping with Anxiety Disorder: How to stop anxiety tension.'

Chapter 1

What is Anxiety Disorder?

Among various human emotions, anxiety is one of the most common emotions. It is an emotional or physical turmoil, which can arise from an event or thoughts. Every person in his or her life experiences anxiety or nervousness in many occasions. Our modern life is full of problems, frustrations, time limits and demands. Arguably, stress is not always bad. A person needs anxiety to some extent; it is required for creativity, learning new things and your survival skills. It helps you to be more focused, energetic and prepared.

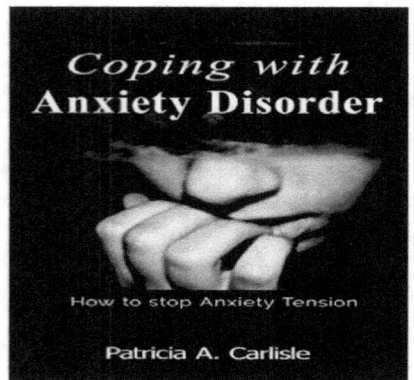

check out the rest of (Coping with Anxiety Disorder: How to stop anxiety tension) on Amazon.

Check Out My Other Books

Below you'll find some of my other popular books that are popular on Amazon and Kindle as well. Alternatively, you can visit my author page on Amazon to see other work done by me.

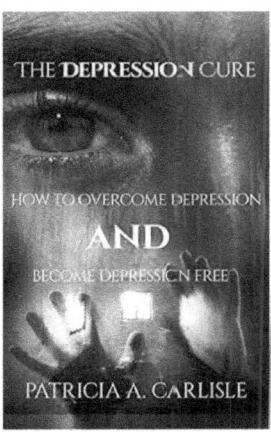

THE DEPRESSION CURE: How to overcome depression and become depression free.

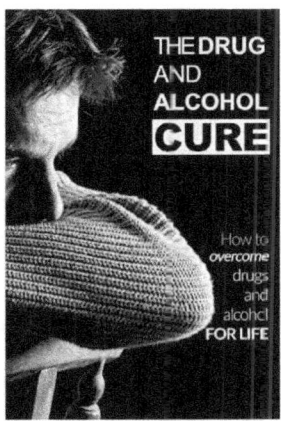

THE DRUG AND ALCOHOL CURE: How to overcome drugs and alcohol for life.

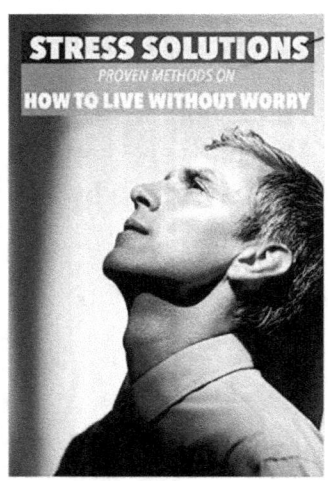

STRESS SOLUTIONS: Proven methods on how to live without worry.

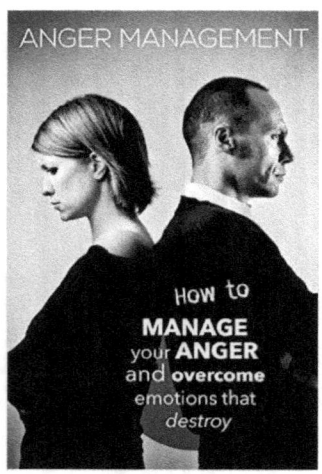

ANGER MANAGEMENT: How to manage your anger and overcome emotions that destroy.

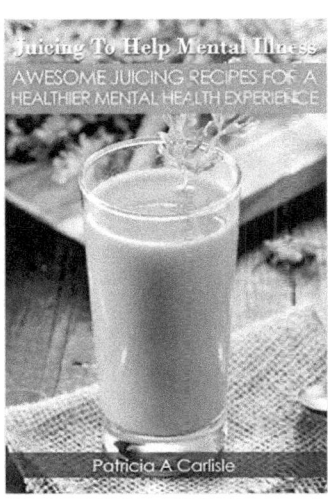

JUICING TO HELP MENTAL ILLNESS: Awesome juicing recipes for a healthier mental health.

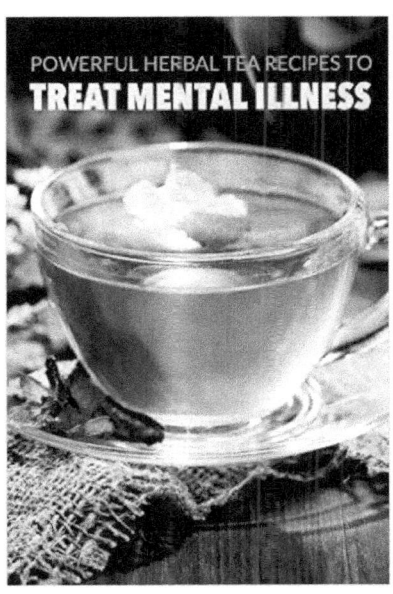

POWERFUL HERBAL TEA RECIPES TO TREAT MENTAL ILLNESS.

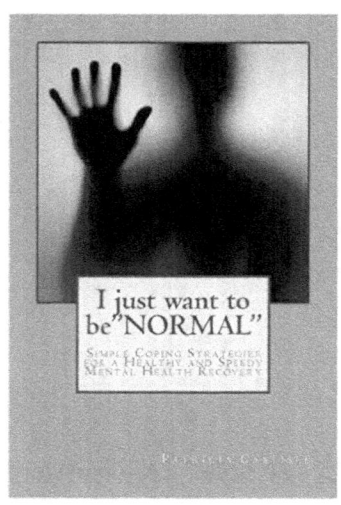

I JUST WANT TO BE "NORMAL" Simple Coping Strategies for a Healthy and Speedy Mental Health Recovery.

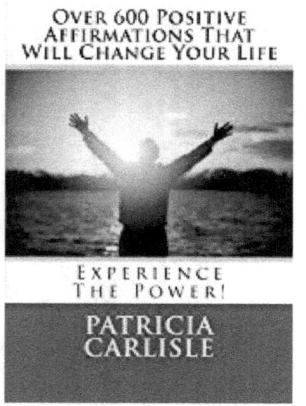

OVER 600 POSITIVE AFFIRMATIONS THAT WILL CHANGE YOUR LIFE: EXPERIENCE THE POWER!

BONUS: SUBSCRIBE TO THE FREE BOOK

Beginners Guide to Yoga & Meditation

"Stressed out? Do You Feel Like The World Is Crashing Down Around You? Want To Take A Vacation That Will Relax Your Mind, Body And Spirit? Well this Easy To Read Step By Step

E-Book Makes It All Possible!"

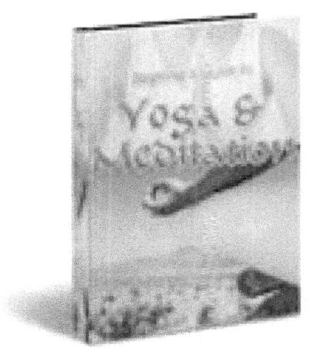

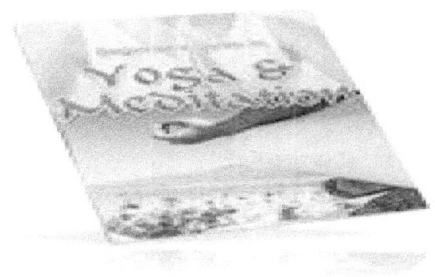

Instructions on how to join our mailing list, and receive a free copy of "Yoga and Meditation" can be found in any of my Kindle eBooks.

NOTE

NOTE

NOTE

NOTE